Step by step Pregnancy Workout Guide

Ultimate pregnancy workout guide for the first time mom with easy routine to help the baby

Jeff Anderson

TABLE OF CONTENT

Chapter 1: Understanding Exercise During Pregnancy: A Comprehensive Overview

Chapter 2: Building a Strong Foundation: Preparing Your Body for Pregnancy Workouts

Chapter 3: Trimester-Specific Workouts: Navigating the Changing Body

Chapter 4: Low-Impact Cardiovascular Exercises: Keeping the Heart Healthy

Chapter 5: Strength Training for a Healthy Pregnancy: Building and Maintaining Muscle Tone

Chapter 6: Mind-Body Connection: Incorporating Prenatal Yoga and Relaxation Techniques

Chapter 7: Special Considerations: Workouts for Common Pregnancy Challenges

Chapter 8: Preparing for Labor and Beyond: The Final Stretch and Postpartum Exercise

Chapter 1

Understanding Exercise During Pregnancy: A Comprehensive Overview

Bringing a new life into the world is a profound journey, and maintaining physical activity during pregnancy can play a crucial role in promoting both maternal and fetal well-being. In this foundational chapter, we embark on a comprehensive exploration of the benefits of staying active during the incredible journey of pregnancy.

Section 1: The Prenatal Advantage

- Delve into the myriad of benefits that regular exercise brings to expectant mothers.

- Discuss how maintaining physical activity during pregnancy can improve mood, reduce the risk of gestational diabetes, and enhance overall mental and emotional well-being.

Section 2: Fetal Benefits of Maternal Exercise

 - Explore the fascinating ways in which a mother's physical activity positively impacts the developing fetus.

 - Discuss the potential long-term benefits for the baby, including improved cardiovascular health and a lower risk of childhood obesity.

Section 3: Mitigating Common Pregnancy Discomforts

- Examine how appropriate exercise can help alleviate common discomforts associated with pregnancy, such as back pain, swelling, and constipation.

- Introduce the idea that tailored workouts can enhance overall comfort and mobility during this transformative time.

Section 4: Maintaining Healthy Weight and Energy Levels

- Discuss the role of exercise in managing weight gain during pregnancy, promoting a healthy balance.

- Explore how staying active contributes to sustained energy levels, combating fatigue and promoting a sense of vitality.

Section 5: Emotional Well-Being and Stress Reduction

- Explore the connection between physical activity and emotional well-being during pregnancy.

- Discuss how exercise can be a powerful tool for stress reduction, anxiety management, and the promotion of a positive mindset.

Section 6: Enhancing Sleep Quality

- Discuss the impact of regular exercise on improving sleep patterns during pregnancy.

- Offer insights into how a consistent fitness routine can contribute to better sleep quality for expectant mothers.

Section 7: Strengthening the Bond Between Mother and Baby

- Highlight the emotional connection that exercise fosters between the mother and the growing baby.

- Discuss the potential psychological benefits of staying active, including a sense of empowerment and connection.

By the end of this chapter, readers will have a profound understanding of the multifaceted benefits that come with staying active during pregnancy. Armed with knowledge, expectant mothers can confidently embark on a journey of wellness, embracing the transformative power of exercise for both themselves and their developing babies.

Navigating the Trimesters: Safety Considerations and Guidelines for Pregnancy Exercise

Embarking on a fitness journey during pregnancy requires a nuanced understanding of the body's changing dynamics across the trimesters. In this chapter, we delve into the essential safety considerations and guidelines that will empower expectant mothers to exercise with confidence, embracing the transformative power of movement while prioritizing maternal and fetal well-being.

Section 1: Safety First - The Importance of Consultation

- Emphasize the paramount importance of consulting with healthcare professionals before initiating any exercise routine during pregnancy.

- Discuss the role of obstetricians, midwives, and other healthcare providers in providing personalized advice based on individual health histories.

Section 2: The First Trimester - Navigating the Early Months

- Explore the considerations and adaptations necessary for safe exercise during the delicate first trimester.

- Discuss common symptoms and challenges, such as morning sickness, and provide suitable modifications for exercise routines.

Section 3: The Second Trimester - Embracing the Midway Mark

- Discuss the physical changes that occur during the second trimester and how they may impact exercise capabilities.

- Introduce guidelines for adapting and modifying workouts to accommodate a growing belly while maintaining intensity and safety.

Section 4: The Third Trimester - Approaching the Finish Line

- Explore the unique challenges and opportunities presented by the third trimester.

- Provide safety considerations for exercises in the later stages of pregnancy, emphasizing the importance of listening to the body.

Section 5: General Guidelines Across Trimesters

- Offer overarching guidelines applicable throughout pregnancy, such as the importance of hydration and avoiding activities with a high risk of falling or abdominal trauma.

- Discuss the significance of paying attention to warning signs and seeking medical advice if any concerns arise.

Section 6: Tailoring Workouts to Individual Comfort and Ability

- Encourage expectant mothers to listen to their bodies and adjust workout intensity and duration based on how they feel.

- Provide guidance on recognizing signs of overexertion and the importance of modifying or stopping exercises accordingly.

Section 7: Pelvic Floor Health - A Focus Throughout Pregnancy

- Discuss the importance of pelvic floor exercises in maintaining strength and integrity during and after pregnancy.

- Provide step-by-step guidance on pelvic floor exercises suitable for each trimester.

By the end of this chapter, readers will have a comprehensive understanding of the safety considerations and guidelines that underpin a healthy and effective pregnancy exercise routine. Empowered with this knowledge, expectant mothers can navigate each trimester with confidence, making informed choices that prioritize the well-being of both themselves and their developing babies.

Navigating the Journey Safely: The Vital Role of Healthcare Consultation in Pregnancy Exercise

Embarking on a fitness journey during pregnancy is a transformative experience, but ensuring the safety and well-being of both mother and baby requires a collaborative effort. This chapter sheds light on the critical importance of consulting with healthcare professionals before initiating any exercise program during pregnancy. It underscores the unique considerations, individual differences, and personalized guidance that healthcare providers bring to the table.

Section 1: The Personalized Pregnancy Experience

- Emphasize that each pregnancy is a unique journey, and the guidance of healthcare professionals is invaluable in tailoring exercise recommendations to individual needs.

- Discuss how factors such as pre-existing medical conditions, previous pregnancy history, and the current health status of the expectant mother contribute to the necessity for personalized advice.

Section 2: The Role of Obstetricians, Midwives, and Healthcare Providers

- Explore the expertise that obstetricians, midwives, and other healthcare providers bring to the realm of pregnancy exercise.

- Discuss the collaborative relationship between the expectant mother and healthcare professionals in ensuring a safe and healthy pregnancy journey.

Section 3: Early Consultation - Setting the Foundation for Fitness

- Advocate for early consultation with healthcare professionals before embarking on any exercise routine.

- Discuss the benefits of establishing an open line of communication, allowing healthcare providers to monitor and guide the expectant mother throughout the entire pregnancy.

Section 4: Addressing Unique Health Considerations

- Highlight the importance of disclosing all relevant health information during consultations.

- Discuss specific health considerations, such as gestational diabetes, hypertension, or musculoskeletal issues, and how they may influence exercise recommendations.

Section 5: Monitoring and Adapting Throughout Pregnancy

- Discuss the dynamic nature of pregnancy and the need for ongoing communication with healthcare providers.

- Emphasize that exercise recommendations may need to be adjusted based on the changing needs of both the mother and the developing baby.

Section 6: Red Flags and Warning Signs

- Provide a list of red flags and warning signs that should prompt immediate consultation with healthcare professionals.

- Stress the importance of seeking guidance if there are any uncertainties or concerns about the safety of specific exercises.

Section 7: The Emotional Support of Healthcare Professionals

- Acknowledge the emotional aspect of pregnancy and how healthcare professionals provide not only physical guidance but also emotional support.

- Encourage expectant mothers to openly discuss any fears, anxieties, or emotional challenges they may face during their fitness journey.

By the end of this chapter, readers will understand that healthcare consultation is not just a precaution but an integral part of a healthy and enjoyable pregnancy exercise experience. The collaborative effort between expectant mothers and healthcare professionals ensures a journey that is not only safe but also empowering, setting the stage for a positive and fulfilling pregnancy.

Chapter 2

Building a Strong Foundation: Preparing Your Body for Pregnancy Workouts

Before embarking on the exhilarating journey of pregnancy workouts, it's essential to lay a solid foundation. This chapter serves as a compass, guiding readers through a comprehensive pre-pregnancy fitness assessment. By understanding their current fitness levels and addressing specific areas, expectant mothers can set the stage for a safe, effective, and enjoyable workout experience during pregnancy.

Section 1: The Significance of Pre-Pregnancy Fitness Assessment

- Introduce the concept of a pre-pregnancy fitness assessment as a crucial starting point for a tailored workout plan.

- Emphasize the role of self-awareness and understanding individual capabilities in promoting a healthy and positive pregnancy exercise experience.

Section 2: Cardiovascular Fitness Evaluation

- Provide guidance on assessing cardiovascular fitness through activities like brisk walking, jogging, or cycling.

- Discuss the importance of a strong cardiovascular foundation in supporting the increased demands of pregnancy.

Section 3: Strength and Muscular Endurance Assessment

- Explore exercises for evaluating strength and muscular endurance, focusing on major muscle groups.

- Discuss the significance of maintaining strength to support the changing body during pregnancy.

Section 4: Flexibility and Joint Mobility Evaluation

- Introduce stretches and exercises for assessing flexibility and joint mobility.

- Emphasize the role of flexibility in preventing discomfort and promoting overall comfort during pregnancy.

Section 5: Core Strength and Stability Analysis

- Discuss the importance of a stable core during pregnancy.

- Introduce exercises that assess core strength and stability, addressing the unique challenges posed by the changing abdominal area.

Section 6: Pelvic Floor Health Assessment

- Explore exercises and techniques to evaluate pelvic floor health.

- Emphasize the crucial role of a strong and well-functioning pelvic floor in preventing issues during and after pregnancy.

Section 7: Assessing Balance and Coordination

- Discuss exercises that evaluate balance and coordination.

- Emphasize their importance in promoting overall stability, reducing the risk of falls, and enhancing comfort during daily activities.

Section 8: Mind-Body Connection: Assessing Stress Levels and Mental Well-Being

- Introduce activities that assess stress levels and mental well-being.

- Discuss the interconnectedness of physical and mental health, emphasizing the holistic approach to pre-pregnancy fitness.

Section 9: Tailoring the Assessment to Individual Needs

- Acknowledge that every expectant mother is unique, requiring a personalized approach to the fitness assessment.

- Provide guidance on modifying exercises based on individual circumstances, encouraging a supportive and inclusive fitness journey.

By the end of this chapter, readers will have conducted a comprehensive pre-pregnancy fitness assessment, gaining valuable insights into their current fitness levels and areas that may need attention. Armed with this knowledge, they can confidently progress to the next chapters, where tailored workout routines will be crafted to meet their individual needs and pave the way for a healthy and fulfilling pregnancy.

Building a Strong Foundation: Preparing Your Body for Pregnancy Workouts

Section 10: Gentle Exercises and Stretches for the Journey Ahead

As you embark on the transformative journey of pregnancy workouts, the significance of preparing your body cannot be overstated. This section introduces a series of gentle exercises and stretches designed to lay the foundation for the physical demands of pregnancy. These activities not only enhance flexibility and strength but also foster a mind-body connection, setting the stage for a healthy and joyful experience.

1. Pelvic Tilts:

- Begin with pelvic tilts, a gentle exercise to engage and strengthen the muscles of the lower back and pelvis.

- Emphasize the importance of controlled movements, promoting awareness of the pelvic region.

2. Cat-Cow Stretch:

- Transition into the cat-cow stretch, a dynamic movement that enhances spinal flexibility.

- Encourage a fluid transition between arching and rounding the back, promoting mobility in the spine.

3. Hip Circles:

- Guide readers through hip circles, promoting flexibility and range of motion in the hip joints.

- Highlight the fluidity of the movement, allowing for a gentle stretch in the hips and lower back.

4. Seated Forward Bend:

- Introduce the seated forward bend to stretch the spine, hamstrings, and lower back.

- Emphasize maintaining a gentle stretch without overexertion, acknowledging individual flexibility levels.

5. Chest Opener Stretch:

- Guide readers through a chest opener stretch to counteract the effects of rounded shoulders.

- Emphasize deep, controlled breathing to enhance relaxation and openness in the chest area.

6. Kegel Exercises:

- Introduce Kegel exercises to strengthen the pelvic floor muscles.

- Discuss the importance of incorporating Kegels into the daily routine for pelvic floor health and support.

7. Modified Plank:

- Ease into a modified plank position to engage the core muscles.

- Emphasize maintaining proper form and adjusting the intensity based on individual comfort levels.

8. Wall Squats:
- Guide readers through wall squats to strengthen the quadriceps, hamstrings, and glutes.
- Emphasize the importance of proper form, including keeping the back straight and knees aligned.

9. Gentle Cardio:
- Introduce low-impact cardiovascular exercises such as walking or swimming.
- Highlight the benefits of cardiovascular fitness in supporting overall health and energy levels during pregnancy.

10. Mindful Breathing:

- Conclude with mindful breathing exercises to promote relaxation and stress reduction.

- Emphasize the connection between breath and movement, fostering a sense of mindfulness and calmness.

By incorporating these gentle exercises and stretches into your routine, you are not only preparing your body for the physical demands of pregnancy but also cultivating a mindful and nurturing approach to your well-being. As you engage in these activities, listen to your body, and embrace the journey ahead with strength, flexibility, and a deep connection to the miraculous process of creating life.

Building a Strong Foundation: Preparing Your Body for Pregnancy Workouts

Section 11: Core and Pelvic Floor Excellence for Stability

In the intricate dance of pregnancy, the core and pelvic floor play starring roles, providing stability and support to your ever-changing body. This section highlights the profound significance of incorporating targeted exercises for the core and pelvic floor into your pre-pregnancy fitness routine. These exercises not only lay the groundwork for a resilient midsection but also promote stability, balance, and overall well-being throughout your pregnancy journey.

1. Understanding the Core:
- Begin by emphasizing the concept of the "core," encompassing not only the abdominal muscles but also the back, pelvis, and diaphragm.
- Discuss how a strong and stable core is the anchor for the body during pregnancy, supporting the growing uterus and minimizing back strain.

2. Pelvic Tilt Exercises:

- Introduce pelvic tilt exercises to engage and strengthen the muscles of the lower back and pelvis.

- Emphasize controlled movements, focusing on the tilting motion that activates both the abdominal and lower back muscles.

3. Modified Planks:

- Transition into modified plank exercises to engage the entire core.

- Discuss the benefits of modified planks in building abdominal strength without undue stress on the lower back.

4. Transverse Abdominis Activation:

- Guide readers through exercises that specifically target the transverse abdominis, a deep abdominal muscle.

- Emphasize the role of the transverse abdominis in providing stability to the spine and pelvis.

5. Pelvic Floor Exercises:

- Introduce pelvic floor exercises, including Kegels, to strengthen the muscles supporting the pelvic organs.

- Discuss the importance of pelvic floor health in preventing issues such as incontinence and supporting the growing uterus during pregnancy.

6. Bridge Exercises:

- Guide readers through bridge exercises to activate the glutes, hamstrings, and lower back while engaging the core.
- Emphasize the controlled lifting of the pelvis, focusing on the engagement of the core and pelvic floor muscles.

7. Leg Raises:
- Introduce leg raises as a gentle exercise to engage the lower abdominal muscles and the hip flexors.
- Discuss modifications for different fitness levels, encouraging gradual progression.

8. Seated Kegels:

- Transition into seated Kegels to provide a different angle for pelvic floor engagement.

- Discuss the importance of incorporating Kegel exercises into daily routines for ongoing pelvic floor health.

9. Yoga Poses for Core and Pelvic Floor:

- Integrate yoga poses such as cat-cow and child's pose to enhance flexibility and promote mindfulness in core and pelvic floor engagement.

- Discuss the holistic benefits of yoga in supporting both physical and mental well-being.

10. The Interconnectedness of Stability:

- Conclude by emphasizing how core and pelvic floor stability are interconnected, forming the foundation for overall body stability.

- Encourage a holistic approach to fitness that considers the synergy of various muscle groups for optimal support.

By incorporating these targeted core and pelvic floor exercises into your pre-pregnancy fitness routine, you are not only fostering stability but also building a resilient foundation for the unique challenges and joys of pregnancy. As you embark on this journey, revel in the strength and stability you are cultivating, laying the groundwork for a healthy and empowered pregnancy experience.

Chapter 3

Trimester-Specific Workouts:

Navigating the Changing Body

Embarking on trimester-specific workouts is a dynamic and empowering approach to pregnancy fitness. This chapter serves as your guide, helping you tailor your workout routines to each trimester while considering the intricate physiological changes your body undergoes. By understanding and embracing these changes, you'll cultivate a fitness routine that not only supports your well-being but also adapts harmoniously to the evolving stages of pregnancy.

Section 1: First Trimester - Laying the Foundation

- Discuss the initial adjustments and adaptations your body undergoes during the first trimester.
- Introduce low-impact cardiovascular exercises and strength training routines tailored to energize without overexerting.

Section 2: Second Trimester - Embracing the Midway Mark

- Explore the increased energy and stability often experienced during the second trimester.

- Introduce modified strength training, flexibility exercises, and low-impact cardio to support the evolving needs of your body.

Section 3: Third Trimester - Nurturing Your Changing Shape

- Address the unique challenges and opportunities presented by the third trimester.

- Introduce gentle exercises, stretches, and modified movements to accommodate your changing body while maintaining strength and flexibility.

Section 4: Cardiovascular Fitness Across Trimesters

- Discuss the importance of maintaining cardiovascular fitness throughout pregnancy.

- Introduce trimester-specific modifications for cardiovascular exercises, ensuring an optimal balance between stamina and comfort.

Section 5: Strength Training Through the Trimesters

- Explore trimester-specific strength training routines, emphasizing modifications to accommodate the changing demands on your muscles.

- Discuss the benefits of maintaining muscle tone for overall strength and support.

Section 6: Flexibility and Stretching Across Trimesters

- Highlight the role of flexibility in promoting comfort and preventing muscle tension.

- Introduce gentle stretching routines tailored to each trimester, focusing on areas prone to tightness.

Section 7: Mind-Body Connection Throughout Pregnancy

- Emphasize the importance of mindfulness and breathing techniques in maintaining a strong mind-body connection.

- Introduce relaxation exercises suitable for each trimester to alleviate stress and promote emotional well-being.

Section 8: Prenatal Yoga and Low-Impact Exercises

- Discuss the benefits of prenatal yoga in promoting flexibility, relaxation, and mental clarity.

- Introduce low-impact exercises suitable for each trimester, ensuring safety and comfort while supporting overall fitness.

Section 9: Listening to Your Body - A Guiding Principle

- Encourage a deep connection with your body, emphasizing the significance of listening to its cues.

- Discuss the importance of modifying or skipping exercises when needed and seeking guidance from healthcare professionals.

By the end of this chapter, you will have a trimester-specific roadmap, ensuring that your workouts evolve in harmony with your changing body. Embrace the adaptability of your fitness routine, revel in the unique strengths each trimester brings, and cultivate a holistic approach to pregnancy fitness that nurtures both your physical and emotional well-being.

Trimester-Specific Workouts: Navigating the Changing Body

Section 10: Step-by-Step Exercises for Each Trimester

Embarking on a trimester-specific workout journey is a testament to your commitment to a healthy and empowered pregnancy. This section provides you with step-by-step exercises carefully curated for each trimester, ensuring that your fitness routine adapts seamlessly to the evolving needs of your changing body.

1. First Trimester: Building a Strong Foundation
Exercise 1: Gentle Cardiovascular Warm-Up
 - Begin with a light cardio warm-up, such as brisk walking or stationary

cycling, to elevate your heart rate gradually.

- Emphasize the importance of a warm-up to prepare your body for exercise.

Exercise 2: Squats with Bodyweight

- Perform squats with a focus on maintaining good form and engaging your glutes.

- Emphasize controlled movements and avoid deep squats to prevent unnecessary strain.

Exercise 3: Seated Rows with Resistance Bands

- Use resistance bands for seated rows to strengthen the upper back muscles.

- Discuss proper posture and breathing techniques during resistance exercises.

2. Second Trimester: Embracing Stability and Energy

Exercise 4: Prenatal Yoga - Cat-Cow Pose

- Introduce the cat-cow pose as part of a prenatal yoga routine to enhance spine flexibility.

- Emphasize the importance of controlled movements and synchronization with breath.

Exercise 5: Side-Lying Leg Lifts for Hip Strength

- Perform side-lying leg lifts to target the hip muscles.

- Discuss modifications based on individual comfort and any existing pelvic discomfort.

Exercise 6: Modified Planks for Core Engagement

- Engage in modified planks to strengthen the core without putting excess pressure on the abdomen.

- Emphasize proper alignment and the importance of engaging the entire core.

3. Third Trimester: Nurturing Your Changing Shape

Exercise 7: Wall Push-Ups for Upper Body Strength

- Utilize wall push-ups to maintain upper body strength while minimizing strain.

- Emphasize keeping the body in a straight line and adjusting the intensity based on comfort.

Exercise 8: Pelvic Tilts for Lower Back Comfort

- Incorporate pelvic tilts to alleviate lower back discomfort.

- Emphasize controlled movements and the benefits of pelvic tilts in promoting comfort.

Exercise 9: Standing Leg Lifts for Balance

- Perform standing leg lifts to enhance balance and target the hip and thigh muscles.

- Discuss the importance of a stable support and gradual movements.

General Tips Across Trimesters:

- Emphasize the significance of staying hydrated and maintaining proper nutrition throughout your workout journey.

- Encourage regular breaks and modifications as needed, allowing for flexibility based on individual comfort levels.

- Discuss the importance of listening to your body, modifying exercises, and seeking professional advice if any discomfort or concerns arise.

By incorporating these step-by-step exercises into your trimester-specific workout routine, you are not only nurturing your physical well-being but also fostering a deep connection with your changing body. Celebrate each trimester as a unique phase, embracing the strength, flexibility, and resilience that these exercises bring to your journey of pregnancy fitness.

Trimester-Specific Workouts: Navigating the Changing Body

Section 11: Embracing Variability - Modifications for Varying Energy Levels

One of the beautiful aspects of pregnancy is the ebb and flow of energy levels. This section acknowledges and celebrates the diversity of energy levels that each trimester brings. By offering modifications and adjustments tailored to varying energy levels and physical capabilities, you can create a workout routine that is both adaptable and empowering.

1. Low-Energy Modifications:
Exercise 1: Seated Cardiovascular Exercises
- Replace high-impact cardio with seated exercises like seated marches or stationary cycling.

- Emphasize the importance of maintaining cardiovascular health while respecting energy limitations.

Exercise 2: Modified Squats with Support

- Perform squats with the support of a chair to reduce the impact on joints.
- Discuss the benefits of maintaining lower body strength while accommodating lower energy levels.

2. Moderate-Energy Adjustments:

Exercise 3: Walking Lunges with Support

- Introduce walking lunges with support to engage the lower body and enhance balance.

- Discuss the option of incorporating lunges without forward motion for added stability.

Exercise 4: Bodyweight Rows on an Incline

- Modify bodyweight rows by performing them on an incline for upper body strength.

- Emphasize controlled movements and proper form while accommodating energy fluctuations.

3. High-Energy Options:

Exercise 5: Dynamic Prenatal Yoga Sequences

- Incorporate dynamic prenatal yoga sequences to enhance flexibility and strength.

- Discuss the benefits of yoga in promoting energy flow and mental clarity for those with higher energy levels.

Exercise 6: Modified Planks with Leg Lifts

- Add leg lifts to modified planks for an extra challenge, targeting core and hip muscles.

- Emphasize the option to skip the leg lifts or reduce the duration based on individual capabilities.

General Tips Across Energy Levels:

- Encourage regular check-ins with your body to gauge energy levels before, during, and after each workout.

- Highlight the importance of setting realistic expectations and adjusting the intensity of exercises accordingly.

- Discuss the potential benefits of incorporating short, frequent workouts to accommodate energy fluctuations throughout the day.

Adjustments for Physical Capabilities:

- Offer seated variations for exercises that may be challenging in a standing position.

- Discuss the option of using resistance bands or bodyweight exercises for those who may need to avoid heavy lifting.

- Emphasize the importance of maintaining a pain-free range of motion and providing alternatives for exercises that may cause discomfort.

By embracing modifications and adjustments that cater to varying energy levels and physical capabilities, you are not only customizing your workout routine but also fostering a sense of inclusivity and self-compassion. This approach ensures that your pregnancy fitness journey is not about pushing boundaries but about honoring and nurturing your body at every stage.

Chapter 4

Low-Impact Cardiovascular Exercises: Keeping the Heart Healthy

Pregnancy brings a unique set of considerations, and maintaining cardiovascular health is paramount for both you and your growing baby. This chapter is dedicated to introducing a curated selection of safe and effective low-impact cardiovascular exercises tailored specifically for pregnant women. By engaging in these heart-healthy workouts, you can foster endurance, support overall well-being, and relish the benefits of cardiovascular fitness during this transformative journey.

Section 1: The Importance of Cardiovascular Health During Pregnancy

- Establish the significance of cardiovascular health for expectant mothers.

- Discuss how maintaining a strong cardiovascular system supports increased blood flow, stamina, and overall vitality during pregnancy.

Section 2: Benefits of Low-Impact Cardiovascular Exercises

- Explore the advantages of low-impact exercises, especially during pregnancy.

- Discuss how these exercises promote cardiovascular fitness without placing excessive stress on joints and ligaments.

Section 3: Walking for Wellness

- Introduce walking as a simple yet effective low-impact cardiovascular exercise.

- Discuss the benefits of brisk walking for heart health, circulation, and mood enhancement.

Section 4: Swimming - Embracing Weightlessness

- Explore the benefits of swimming as a low-impact cardiovascular exercise.

- Discuss how the buoyancy of water reduces strain on joints, making it an ideal choice for pregnant women.

Section 5: Stationary Cycling - Pedaling for Health

- Introduce stationary cycling as a safe and effective way to elevate heart rate.
- Discuss the benefits of cycling, emphasizing the controlled nature of stationary bikes.

Section 6: Prenatal Aerobics - Tailored for Pregnancy

- Discuss the concept of prenatal aerobics and its focus on low-impact movements.

- Introduce gentle aerobics routines designed to boost cardiovascular fitness while accommodating the changing body.

Section 7: Elliptical Training - Smooth Strides for Strength

- Explore elliptical training as a low-impact alternative to traditional running.

- Discuss the benefits of elliptical machines in providing a full-body workout with minimal impact.

Section 8: Low-Impact Dance Workouts - Grooving Safely

- Introduce low-impact dance workouts tailored for pregnancy.

- Discuss the enjoyment and cardiovascular benefits of dancing while emphasizing safety and comfort.

Section 9: Safety Considerations and Precautions

- Provide essential safety guidelines for engaging in low-impact cardiovascular exercises during pregnancy.

- Discuss the importance of consulting with healthcare professionals before starting or modifying any exercise routine.

Section 10: Crafting a Personalized Cardiovascular Routine

- Encourage readers to tailor their cardiovascular routines based on individual preferences, fitness levels, and energy levels.

- Discuss the flexibility of combining different exercises for variety and sustained motivation.

By the end of this chapter, expectant mothers will have a comprehensive understanding of the importance of cardiovascular health during pregnancy and a diverse set of low-impact exercises to choose from. These heart-healthy workouts are not only safe and effective but also contribute to an enjoyable and fulfilling pregnancy fitness routine.

Low-Impact Cardiovascular Exercises: Keeping the Heart Healthy

Section 11: The Dual Triumph - Benefits for Both Mother and Baby

Embarking on a journey of low-impact cardiovascular exercises during pregnancy extends beyond personal well-being. This section delves into the remarkable benefits that these heart-healthy workouts bestow not only upon the expectant mother but also upon the growing baby within, fostering a symbiotic relationship that nurtures health and vitality.

1. Enhanced Cardiovascular Fitness for the Mother:

Benefit 1: Improved Circulation

- Discuss how low-impact cardiovascular exercises enhance blood circulation.

- Emphasize the positive impact on oxygen and nutrient delivery to both the mother's body and the developing baby.

Benefit 2: Increased Stamina and Endurance

- Explore how regular cardiovascular workouts improve stamina and endurance.

- Discuss the relevance of heightened endurance during labor and delivery, contributing to a smoother birthing experience.

Benefit 3: Mood Elevation and Stress Reduction

- Highlight the mood-boosting effects of cardiovascular exercises through the release of endorphins.

- Discuss how managing stress positively impacts the mental and emotional well-being of the expectant mother.

Benefit 4: Weight Management and Energy Levels

- Discuss the role of cardiovascular workouts in supporting healthy weight management during pregnancy.

- Emphasize how sustained energy levels contribute to an active and fulfilling lifestyle.

2. Nurturing Development for the Growing Baby:

Benefit 1: Improved Placental Function

- Explore how maternal cardiovascular health positively influences placental function.

- Discuss the importance of the placenta in supplying essential nutrients and oxygen to the growing baby.

Benefit 2: Potential for Enhanced Fetal Brain Development

- Introduce studies suggesting a potential link between maternal cardiovascular fitness and enhanced fetal brain development.

- Discuss the implications of optimal oxygen and nutrient supply for the developing baby's neurological health.

Benefit 3: Potential Reduction in Fetal Stress Responses

- Discuss research indicating that regular maternal exercise may contribute to a reduction in fetal stress responses.

- Explore the potential long-term benefits for the baby's stress resilience.

Benefit 4: Healthy Birth Weight and Overall Well-Being

- Explore how maintaining cardiovascular health may contribute to a healthy birth weight for the baby.

- Discuss the potential correlation between maternal fitness and the overall well-being of the newborn.

3. Bonding Through Shared Well-Being:

- Emphasize how the shared experience of low-impact cardiovascular exercises can foster a unique bond between the mother and the growing baby.

- Discuss the joy and sense of connection that comes from engaging in activities that benefit both parties.

4. Safety and Moderation:

- Reiterate the importance of consulting with healthcare professionals before starting or modifying any exercise routine during pregnancy.

- Emphasize the need for moderation and gradual progression, ensuring the safety and well-being of both the mother and the baby.

By understanding and embracing the dual triumph of benefits that cardiovascular workouts bring to both the mother and the baby, expectant mothers can embark on a journey that goes beyond personal fitness—a journey that nurtures the health and vitality of the entire family unit.

Low-Impact Cardiovascular Exercises: Keeping the Heart Healthy

Section 12: Versatility in Motion - Indoor and Outdoor Cardiovascular Activities for All Fitness Levels

The beauty of cardiovascular exercises lies in their adaptability to various environments and fitness levels. This section explores a diverse array of indoor and outdoor activities tailored for pregnant women, ensuring inclusivity and flexibility in maintaining heart health. Whether you prefer the comfort of your home or the embrace of nature, there's a low-impact exercise suitable for every fitness level.

1. Indoor Cardiovascular Activities:

Option 1: Home-Based Aerobics:

- Explore low-impact aerobics routines that can be performed in the comfort of your living room.

- Discuss the convenience of following online prenatal aerobics classes, providing guidance for proper form and technique.

Option 2: Stationary Cycling at Home:

- Introduce stationary cycling as an indoor option, utilizing a stationary bike.

- Discuss the benefits of stationary cycling, including improved cardiovascular health and lower impact on joints.

Option 3: Dance Workouts in a Controlled Environment:

- Recommend low-impact dance workouts suitable for indoor settings.

- Emphasize the joy and cardiovascular benefits of dancing while accommodating different fitness levels.

2. Outdoor Cardiovascular Activities:

Option 4: Brisk Walking in Nature:

 - Encourage brisk walking in outdoor settings such as parks or nature trails.

 - Discuss the benefits of connecting with nature, promoting mental well-being alongside cardiovascular fitness.

Option 5: Swimming in Pools or Calm Waters:

 - Highlight swimming as a serene outdoor option, whether in a pool or calm natural waters.

 - Emphasize the buoyancy of water and its gentle impact on joints.

Option 6: Low-Impact Cycling in Scenic Routes:

- Recommend low-impact cycling in scenic outdoor routes.

- Discuss the benefits of cycling, including improved cardiovascular fitness and the joy of exploring new environments.

3. Adaptations for Different Fitness Levels:

Adaptation 1: Interval Training for Varied Intensity:

- Introduce interval training, allowing individuals to adjust the intensity based on their fitness levels.

- Discuss the benefits of interval training in promoting cardiovascular health while accommodating different energy levels.

Adaptation 2: Seated Cardiovascular Exercises:

-    Provide options for seated cardiovascular exercises for individuals with lower mobility or energy levels.

- Discuss how seated exercises can still contribute to heart health.

Adaptation 3: Incorporating Rest Breaks:

-    Discuss the importance of incorporating rest breaks during cardiovascular activities.

- Emphasize that regular breaks enhance safety, allowing individuals to modify activities based on their comfort.

4. Personalization for Varied Preferences:

- Encourage individuals to personalize their cardiovascular routine based on preferences.

- Discuss how incorporating activities that align with personal interests enhances adherence to fitness goals.

By providing a range of indoor and outdoor options adaptable to different fitness levels, this section empowers expectant mothers to curate a cardiovascular routine that resonates with their preferences, ensuring an enjoyable and inclusive approach to heart-healthy living during pregnancy.

Chapter 5

Strength Training for a Healthy Pregnancy: Building and Maintaining Muscle Tone

Strength training during pregnancy is a powerful ally, providing myriad benefits for both the expectant mother and the growing baby. This chapter serves as a comprehensive guide, leading readers through a series of safe and effective strength training exercises specifically tailored for pregnancy. Embrace the transformative journey of building and maintaining muscle tone to enhance overall well-being and prepare the body for the incredible feat of childbirth.

Section 1: The Benefits of Strength Training During Pregnancy
- Establish the significance of strength training in promoting overall health and fitness.
- Discuss how maintaining muscle tone contributes to improved posture, reduced discomfort, and enhanced stamina during pregnancy.

Section 2: Safety Considerations and Guidelines

- Provide essential safety guidelines for engaging in strength training during pregnancy.

- Emphasize the importance of consulting with healthcare professionals before starting or modifying any exercise routine.

Section 3: Core-Strengthening Exercises for Stability

- Introduce core-strengthening exercises suitable for pregnancy.

- Discuss the importance of a stable core in supporting the growing uterus and reducing strain on the lower back.

Exercise 1: Pelvic Tilts for Core Activation

- Guide readers through pelvic tilts to engage and strengthen the muscles of the lower back and pelvis.

- Emphasize controlled movements and the benefits of pelvic tilts for core stability.

Exercise 2: Modified Planks for Abdominal Strength

- Introduce modified planks to engage the entire core without excessive pressure on the abdomen.

- Discuss variations and the importance of proper form during plank exercises.

Section 4: Upper Body Strength for Daily Activities

- Explore upper body strength training exercises that prepare the body for the physical demands of daily activities.

- Discuss the relevance of maintaining upper body strength for lifting, carrying, and overall functional movement.

Exercise 3: Seated Rows with Resistance Bands

- Demonstrate seated rows using resistance bands to target the upper back muscles.

- Discuss the controlled nature of resistance band exercises and their adaptability for different fitness levels.

Exercise 4: Modified Push-Ups for Arm and Chest Strength

- Guide readers through modified push-ups to strengthen the arms and chest.

- Discuss proper form and provide options for adjusting the intensity based on individual capabilities.

Section 5: Lower Body Strengthening for Stability

- Introduce lower body strength training exercises that enhance stability and support the changing body during pregnancy.

- Discuss the importance of strong lower body muscles for balance and mobility.

Exercise 5: Bodyweight Squats for Leg Strength

- Demonstrate bodyweight squats to target the muscles of the thighs and glutes.

- Emphasize proper squatting technique and the controlled lowering and rising movements.

Exercise 6: Standing Leg Lifts for Balance

- Guide readers through standing leg lifts to engage the hip and thigh muscles.

- Discuss the importance of balance exercises for stability during pregnancy.

Section 6: Flexibility and Warm-Up Exercises

- Highlight the significance of incorporating flexibility exercises and warm-ups before strength training.

- Discuss dynamic stretches and movements to prepare the muscles for the demands of strength training.

Exercise 7: Arm Circles and Shoulder Rolls for Warm-Up

- Introduce arm circles and shoulder rolls as effective warm-up exercises for the upper body.

- Discuss the benefits of improving shoulder mobility and flexibility.

Exercise 8: Leg Swings and Ankle Rolls for Lower Body Warm-Up

- Guide readers through leg swings and ankle rolls to warm up the lower body.

- Discuss how dynamic lower body warm-up exercises enhance flexibility and reduce the risk of injury.

Section 7: Listening to Your Body - A Guiding Principle

- Reiterate the importance of listening to the body during strength training.

- Discuss the significance of modifying or skipping exercises when needed and seeking professional advice if any discomfort or concerns arise.

By guiding readers through these carefully selected strength training exercises, this chapter aims to empower expectant mothers to embrace the benefits of building and maintaining muscle tone during pregnancy. Strengthening the body lays a robust foundation for the challenges and joys that lie ahead, fostering a sense of resilience and empowerment throughout the transformative journey of pregnancy.

Strength Training for a Healthy Pregnancy: Building and Maintaining Muscle Tone

Section 8: Targeted Strength Training - Addressing Common Pregnancy Discomforts

Pregnancy is a beautiful journey, yet it comes with its share of unique physical challenges. This section delves into the importance of targeted strength training, emphasizing exercises that specifically address common discomforts experienced during pregnancy. By strategically focusing on specific muscle groups, expectant mothers can alleviate discomfort, enhance overall well-being, and nurture a stronger connection with their changing bodies.

1. Relieving Lower Back Pain:
Exercise 1: Pelvic Tilts for Lumbar Support

- Highlight pelvic tilts as a targeted exercise to strengthen the muscles supporting the lower back.

- Discuss the role of pelvic tilts in promoting lumbar stability and alleviating lower back pain.

Exercise 2: Cat-Cow Stretch for Spinal Mobility

- Introduce the cat-cow stretch to enhance spinal mobility and flexibility.

- Discuss the benefits of this yoga-inspired movement in relieving tension in the lower back.

2. Easing Hip Discomfort:

Exercise 3: Standing Hip Abduction for Hip Strength

- Guide readers through standing hip abduction exercises to strengthen the muscles around the hips.

- Discuss the role of hip abduction in relieving hip discomfort and enhancing stability.

Exercise 4: Seated Butterfly Stretch for Hip Flexibility

- Introduce the seated butterfly stretch to improve hip flexibility and reduce tightness.

- Discuss how this stretch targets the inner thighs and hip flexors, common areas of discomfort during pregnancy.

3. Alleviating Round Ligament Pain:

Exercise 5: Leg Lifts in Side-Lying Position for Round Ligament Support

 - Demonstrate leg lifts in a side-lying position to target the muscles supporting the round ligaments.

 - Discuss the role of these exercises in providing support to the round ligaments and minimizing pain.

Exercise 6: Gentle Rotational Exercises for Round Ligament Relief

 - Introduce gentle rotational exercises to alleviate round ligament discomfort.

 - Emphasize controlled movements to avoid strain and enhance the flexibility of the torso.

4. Strengthening Pelvic Floor Muscles:

Exercise 7: Kegel Exercises for Pelvic Floor Strength

- Highlight the importance of Kegel exercises in strengthening the pelvic floor muscles.

- Discuss the benefits of Kegels in preventing issues such as incontinence and supporting the growing uterus.

Exercise 8: Squats for Overall Pelvic Stability

- Guide readers through squats to engage multiple muscle groups, including the pelvic floor.

- Discuss how squats contribute to overall pelvic stability and strength.

5. Enhancing Posture and Core Stability:

Exercise 9: Seated Rows for Postural Support

- Demonstrate seated rows using resistance bands to target the muscles of the upper back.

- Discuss the role of these exercises in promoting postural support and reducing strain on the spine.

Exercise 10: Modified Planks for Core Stability

- Revisit modified planks as a core-strengthening exercise.

- Emphasize the importance of a strong core in maintaining good posture and reducing discomfort.

6. Supporting Overall Comfort and Functionality:

Exercise 11: Arm and Shoulder Exercises for Upper Body Strength

- Explore arm and shoulder exercises to enhance overall upper body strength.

- Discuss the relevance of strong upper body muscles for daily activities and functional movement.

Exercise 12: Leg Exercises for General Strength

- Guide readers through leg exercises like bodyweight squats and leg lifts to support overall lower body strength.

- Discuss the holistic benefits of maintaining strength in the legs for stability and functionality.

7. Incorporating Mindful Breathing Techniques:

- Introduce the practice of mindful breathing during strength training exercises.

- Discuss the benefits of conscious breathing in promoting relaxation, reducing tension, and enhancing the mind-body connection.

By focusing on targeted strength training exercises for specific muscle groups, expectant mothers can proactively address common discomforts associated with pregnancy. This targeted approach not only fosters physical well-being but also instills a sense of empowerment as women navigate the beautiful journey of pregnancy with strength, resilience, and mindful awareness.

Strength Training for a Healthy Pregnancy: Building and Maintaining Muscle Tone

Section 9: Adapting Traditions - Modified Strength Training Moves for Safety and Effectiveness

In the realm of strength training during pregnancy, adaptability is key. This section serves as a compass, guiding expectant mothers through modifications of traditional strength training moves, ensuring both safety and effectiveness. By embracing these tailored adjustments, readers can confidently navigate their strength training journey, reaping the benefits without compromising the well-being of themselves or their growing babies.

1. Squats:

Traditional Move: Bodyweight Squats

 - Discuss the benefits of squats for lower body strength and overall stability.

 - Introduce modifications such as shallower squats or using a stable support for balance.

2. Lunges:

Traditional Move: Forward Lunges

- Highlight the importance of lunges for targeting the thighs and glutes.

- Introduce modifications, such as static lunges or reducing the range of motion, to accommodate comfort levels.

3. Deadlifts:

Traditional Move: Romanian Deadlifts with Dumbbells

- Discuss the benefits of deadlifts for the posterior chain.

- Introduce modifications like using lighter weights or performing the movement with bodyweight only.

4. Planks:

Traditional Move: Front Planks

- Emphasize the significance of planks for core strength.

- Introduce modifications such as inclined planks or performing planks on hands and knees to reduce pressure on the abdomen.

5. Push-Ups:

Traditional Move: Standard Push-Ups

- Discuss the benefits of push-ups for upper body strength.

- Introduce modifications, such as performing push-ups against a stable surface or opting for wall push-ups.

6. Rows:

Traditional Move: Bent-Over Rows with Dumbbells

- Highlight the importance of rows for targeting the upper back muscles.

- Introduce modifications like seated rows with resistance bands to minimize strain on the lower back.

7. Shoulder Press:

Traditional Move: Overhead Shoulder Press with Weights

- Discuss the benefits of shoulder presses for upper body strength.

- Introduce modifications like seated shoulder presses or using lighter weights to ensure shoulder stability.

8. Leg Press:

Traditional Move: Leg Press Machine

- Discuss the benefits of leg presses for lower body strength.

- Introduce modifications such as bodyweight leg presses or using resistance bands for a controlled alternative.

9. Bicep Curls:

Traditional Move: Bicep Curls with Dumbbells

- Emphasize the importance of bicep curls for arm strength.

- Introduce modifications such as using lighter weights or incorporating isometric holds for controlled resistance.

10. Tricep Dips:

Traditional Move: Bench Tricep Dips

 - Discuss the benefits of tricep dips for arm strength.

 - Introduce modifications such as chair dips or using stable surfaces for support.

11. Kettlebell Swings:
Traditional Move: Kettlebell Swings

 - Highlight the benefits of kettlebell swings for full-body engagement.

 - Introduce modifications such as bodyweight swings or using lighter kettlebells with controlled movements.

12. Leg Raises:
Traditional Move: Straight Leg Raises

 - Discuss the benefits of leg raises for core strength.

- Introduce modifications like bent-knee leg raises to reduce strain on the lower back.

13. Wall Sits:
Traditional Move: Wall Sits

- Emphasize the benefits of wall sits for lower body endurance.

- Introduce modifications such as partial wall sits or reducing the duration based on individual comfort.

By providing adaptations to traditional strength training moves, this section empowers expectant mothers to customize their workout routine, ensuring a safe and effective journey towards building and maintaining muscle tone during pregnancy. These modifications embrace individual comfort levels, promoting confidence and well-being as women navigate the transformative experience of pregnancy with strength and resilience.

Chapter 6

Mind-Body Connection: Incorporating Prenatal Yoga and Relaxation Techniques

Section 1: The Serene Dance of Body and Mind - Benefits of Prenatal Yoga

Embarking on the journey of pregnancy is not just a physical transformation but a profound connection between the body and mind. Prenatal yoga emerges as a graceful companion, offering a sanctuary for expectant mothers to foster flexibility, find relaxation, and nurture their mental well-being. This chapter delves into the tranquil world of prenatal yoga, unveiling the myriad benefits it bestows upon both the body and the spirit during this transformative period.

1. Nurturing Physical Flexibility:
- Explore how prenatal yoga embraces gentle stretches and poses to enhance overall flexibility.
- Discuss the significance of improved flexibility in easing common physical discomforts associated with pregnancy.

2. Cultivating Relaxation and Stress Relief:

- Highlight the role of mindful breathing and relaxation techniques within prenatal yoga.

- Discuss how these practices contribute to stress reduction, promoting a sense of calmness and tranquility.

3. Enhancing Circulation and Blood Flow:

- Delve into the benefits of prenatal yoga in improving circulation and blood flow.

- Discuss how enhanced blood flow supports the delivery of nutrients and oxygen to both the mother and the developing baby.

4. Alleviating Common Pregnancy Discomforts:

- Explore specific yoga poses tailored to alleviate discomforts such as back pain and swelling.

- Discuss the gentle and therapeutic nature of these poses in promoting physical comfort.

5. Promoting Mindful Connection with the Baby:

- Discuss how prenatal yoga fosters a mindful connection between the mother and the growing baby.

- Explore guided practices that encourage expectant mothers to embrace and celebrate the miracle of life within.

6. Preparing for Labor and Birth:

- Explore the role of prenatal yoga in preparing the body for labor and childbirth.

- Discuss specific poses and movements that aid in building strength and flexibility essential for the birthing process.

7. Fostering Emotional Well-Being:

- Highlight the impact of prenatal yoga on emotional well-being.

- Discuss how the mind-body connection cultivated through yoga contributes to a positive and empowered emotional state.

8. Building a Supportive Community:

- Emphasize the communal aspect of prenatal yoga classes, providing a space for mothers to connect and share their experiences.

- Discuss the sense of support and camaraderie that arises from participating in a community of expectant mothers.

9. Embracing Mindfulness Beyond the Mat:

- Encourage the integration of mindfulness practices learned in prenatal yoga into daily life.

- Discuss how mindfulness contributes to a more present and fulfilling experience of pregnancy.

10. Guided Relaxation Techniques:

- Introduce specific relaxation techniques, such as progressive muscle relaxation and guided imagery.

- Discuss their efficacy in promoting deep relaxation and mental clarity.

By exploring the multifaceted benefits of prenatal yoga, this chapter aims to guide expectant mothers toward a serene and mindful pregnancy journey. Prenatal yoga becomes not just a series of poses but a holistic practice that nurtures the body, soothes the mind, and celebrates the profound connection between a mother and her unborn child.

Mind-Body Connection: Incorporating Prenatal Yoga and Relaxation Techniques

Section 2: The Breath of Calm - Breathing Exercises and Mindfulness Techniques for Stress Reduction

In the rhythmic dance between body and mind, the breath serves as a guiding force, a constant companion through the journey of pregnancy. This section delves into the art of conscious breathing and mindfulness techniques within prenatal yoga, unveiling their transformative power in reducing stress, fostering tranquility, and enhancing the mind-body connection.

1. The Foundation: Diaphragmatic Breathing

- Introduce diaphragmatic breathing as the foundational breathwork technique.

- Discuss the significance of breathing deeply into the diaphragm to promote relaxation and alleviate tension.

2. Equal-Length Breathing: Sama Vritti

- Explore the practice of equal-length breathing, or Sama Vritti, as a balancing breath technique.

- Discuss how inhaling and exhaling for an equal duration calms the nervous system and brings about a sense of equilibrium.

3. Guided Visualization and Breath Awareness

- Introduce guided visualization techniques accompanied by intentional breath awareness.

- Discuss how visualizing calming scenes or focusing on the breath promotes mindfulness, reducing stress and anxiety.

4. Box Breathing: Sama Vritti with Holds

- Explore box breathing, incorporating holds between inhales and exhales.

- Discuss how this technique enhances breath control, deepens relaxation, and encourages a meditative state.

5. Mindful Body Scan

- Introduce the mindful body scan as a technique to promote awareness of physical sensations.

- Discuss how systematically scanning and releasing tension from different parts of the body contributes to overall relaxation.

6. Ocean Breathing: Ujjayi Pranayama

- Explore Ujjayi Pranayama, or ocean breathing, as a technique to create a soothing sound with the breath.

- Discuss the benefits of this rhythmic breath in calming the mind and enhancing focus during yoga practice.

7. Progressive Muscle Relaxation

- Introduce progressive muscle relaxation as a method to release physical tension.

- Discuss the systematic tensing and relaxing of muscle groups, promoting a sense of calmness and ease.

8. Loving-Kindness Meditation: Metta

- Explore loving-kindness meditation, or Metta, as a mindfulness technique.

- Discuss how cultivating feelings of love and compassion towards oneself and others contributes to emotional well-being.

9. Mindful Walking Meditation

- Introduce mindful walking as a form of meditation, synchronizing breath with movement.

- Discuss how this practice fosters a connection between the body and the present moment, reducing stress and promoting clarity.

10. Incorporating Mindfulness into Daily Life
- Encourage the integration of mindfulness techniques into daily routines.
- Discuss how simple practices like mindful breathing during daily activities contribute to sustained stress reduction.

Incorporating these breathing exercises and mindfulness techniques into prenatal yoga not only enriches the practice but becomes a lifeline for expectant mothers navigating the beautiful yet sometimes challenging landscape of pregnancy. Through the mindful cultivation of the breath, the mind-body connection blossoms, creating a sanctuary of peace, resilience, and empowerment during this transformative journey.

Mind-Body Connection: Incorporating Prenatal Yoga and Relaxation Techniques

Section 3: Nurturing the Blossom - Step-by-Step Prenatal Yoga Routines for Different Stages of Pregnancy

Embarking on a prenatal yoga journey is a deeply personal and transformative experience. This section unfolds step-by-step yoga routines tailored for different stages of pregnancy, guiding expectant mothers through a graceful sequence that nurtures their changing bodies, enhances flexibility, and cultivates a profound mind-body connection.

1. First Trimester: Planting the Seeds of Serenity

Pose 1: Mountain Pose (Tadasana)

- Guide readers through Mountain Pose, fostering grounding and stability.

- Emphasize the importance of connecting with the breath while standing tall.

Pose 2: Cat-Cow Stretch (Marjaryasana-Bitilasana)

- Introduce the gentle flow of Cat-Cow Stretch to enhance spinal flexibility.

- Emphasize the synchronized movement with breath, promoting a sense of fluidity.

Pose 3: Supported Warrior II (Virabhadrasana II with Support)

- Guide expectant mothers through a supported version of Warrior II for strength and balance.

- Discuss the use of props for added stability and comfort.

2. Second Trimester: Blossoming into Grace

Pose 4: Goddess Pose (Utkata Konasana)

- Explore Goddess Pose to strengthen the lower body and open the hips.

- Discuss modifications to accommodate comfort and encourage stability.

Pose 5: Prenatal Sun Salutations (Surya Namaskar)

- Introduce a modified version of Sun Salutations for a gentle full-body workout.

- Emphasize fluid movements and the incorporation of breath throughout the sequence.

Pose 6: Seated Pigeon Pose (Eka Pada Rajakapotasana)

- Guide readers through a seated variation of Pigeon Pose for hip opening.

- Discuss the use of props to support proper alignment and ease.

3. Third Trimester: Blooming in Strength and Serenity

Pose 7: Supported Tree Pose (Vrksasana with Support)

- Explore a supported version of Tree Pose to enhance balance.

- Discuss the option of using a chair or wall for added stability.

Pose 8: Modified Bridge Pose (Setu Bandhasana)

- Guide expectant mothers through a modified Bridge Pose for gentle back strengthening.

- Discuss the importance of engaging the core and pelvic floor muscles.

Pose 9: Child's Pose (Balasana) with Props

- Introduce a supported version of Child's Pose for relaxation.

- Discuss the use of props to provide comfort and reduce pressure on the abdomen.

4. Connecting Mind and Body: Mindfulness Meditation for All Trimesters

Mindfulness Meditation: Seated Comfortably with Breath Awareness

- Introduce a seated mindfulness meditation suitable for all trimesters.

- Guide expectant mothers in cultivating awareness of breath and sensations.

5. Closing Sequence: Restorative Poses for Relaxation

Restorative Pose 1: Supported Savasana (Corpse Pose)

- Guide readers through a supported version of Savasana for deep relaxation.

- Discuss the use of props to create a comfortable and nurturing environment.

Restorative Pose 2: Reclining Bound Angle Pose (Supta Baddha Konasana)

- Introduce a restorative version of Bound Angle Pose for hip opening and relaxation.

- Emphasize the importance of surrendering into the pose and releasing tension.

Restorative Pose 3: Side-Lying Shavasana (Corpse Pose)

- Guide expectant mothers through a side-lying variation of Savasana for comfort.

- Discuss the relaxation benefits of this pose, allowing for a gentle release of tension.

By offering these step-by-step yoga routines for each stage of pregnancy, this section aims to provide a thoughtful and nurturing guide for expectant mothers. Each pose and sequence is designed to celebrate the beauty of pregnancy, honoring the body's journey with grace, strength, and the embrace of serene mindfulness.

Chapter 7

Special Considerations: Workouts for Common Pregnancy Challenges

Section 1: Empowering Through Adversity - Tailored Workouts for Common Pregnancy Discomforts

Pregnancy is a miraculous journey, but it comes with its own set of challenges. This chapter addresses common discomforts such as back pain, swelling, and fatigue, providing empowering workouts designed to alleviate these issues. Through mindful exercises, gentle stretches, and targeted movements, expectant mothers can navigate the challenges of pregnancy with strength, resilience, and a renewed sense of well-being.

1. Alleviating Back Pain: Strengthening the Core

Exercise 1: Pelvic Tilts for Lumbar Support

- Guide readers through pelvic tilts to engage and strengthen the muscles supporting the lower back.

- Discuss the importance of these exercises in promoting lumbar stability and alleviating back pain.

Exercise 2: Modified Cat-Cow Stretch for Spinal Comfort

- Introduce a modified Cat-Cow Stretch to gently mobilize the spine and reduce back discomfort.

- Discuss the controlled movements and the benefits of this stretch for easing tension in the lower back.

Exercise 3: Seated Rows with Resistance Bands for Upper Back Support

- Demonstrate seated rows using resistance bands to target the upper back muscles.

- Discuss how strengthening the upper back contributes to overall postural support, reducing strain on the lower back.

2. Managing Swelling: Elevating Leg Exercises

Exercise 4: Seated Leg Lifts for Improved Circulation

- Guide expectant mothers through seated leg lifts to enhance circulation and reduce swelling.

- Discuss the importance of controlled movements and ankle rotations to promote blood flow.

Exercise 5: Ankle Circles and Toe Taps for Fluid Drainage

- Introduce ankle circles and toe taps as exercises to encourage fluid drainage.

- Discuss the benefits of these gentle movements in mitigating swelling, especially in the lower extremities.

Exercise 6: Supported Legs Up the Wall Pose (Viparita Karani) for Relaxation

- Guide readers through a supported version of Legs Up the Wall Pose to alleviate swelling and promote relaxation.

- Discuss the use of props and the calming effects of this inversion on the circulatory system.

3. Combating Fatigue: Energizing Full-Body Movements

Exercise 7: Gentle Cardiovascular Routine for Energy Boost

- Introduce a gentle cardiovascular routine, such as walking or stationary cycling, to combat fatigue.

- Discuss the importance of low-impact exercises for maintaining energy levels without overexertion.

Exercise 8: Seated Marching and Arm Circles for Midday Rejuvenation

- Guide expectant mothers through seated marching and arm circles for a quick midday energy boost.

- Discuss the invigorating effects of these movements on the cardiovascular system.

Exercise 9: Mindful Breathing Breaks for Mental Refreshment

- Introduce short mindful breathing exercises to be incorporated throughout the day.

- Discuss how intentional breathing can provide mental clarity, reduce stress, and combat fatigue.

4. Adapting Workouts for Each Trimester: Progressive Approaches

Trimester 1: Gentle Introduction to Exercise

- Provide a set of beginner-friendly exercises suitable for the first trimester.

- Discuss the importance of gradually incorporating movement into the routine.

Trimester 2: Building Strength and Flexibility

- Introduce slightly more challenging exercises focused on strength and flexibility for the second trimester.

- Discuss modifications and adaptations based on individual comfort levels.

Trimester 3: Mindful Maintenance and Preparation for Birth

- Offer exercises that focus on maintaining energy, mobility, and mental well-being during the third trimester.

- Discuss the importance of listening to the body and preparing for the birthing process through specific movements.

By addressing common pregnancy challenges with tailored workouts, this section aims to empower expectant mothers to embrace their changing bodies with confidence and resilience. Each exercise is thoughtfully designed to provide relief, enhance well-being, and foster a sense of strength, making the journey through pregnancy a more joyous and empowering experience.

Special Considerations: Workouts for Common Pregnancy Challenges

Section 2: Targeted Relief - Exercises and Stretches to Alleviate Specific Challenges

Pregnancy brings a myriad of unique challenges, and this section is dedicated to offering targeted exercises and stretches tailored to alleviate specific discomforts. By focusing on key areas such as back pain, swelling, and muscle fatigue, these exercises empower expectant mothers to address these challenges with precision, promoting a more comfortable and joyful pregnancy experience.

1. Relieving Back Pain: A Therapeutic Sequence

Exercise 1: Child's Pose with Gentle Rocking

 - Guide readers through Child's Pose with gentle rocking to release tension in the lower back.

- Emphasize the soothing effects of rhythmic movement and controlled breathing.

Exercise 2: Seated Spinal Twist (Ardha Matsyendrasana) Modifications

- Demonstrate seated spinal twists with modifications to ease tension in the spine.

- Discuss the importance of maintaining a comfortable seated position and adapting the twist based on individual comfort.

Exercise 3: Pelvic Floor Exercises for Lumbar Support

- Introduce pelvic floor exercises to strengthen the muscles supporting the lower back.

- Discuss the role of a strong pelvic floor in promoting lumbar stability and reducing back pain.

2. Managing Swelling: Limb Elevation and Circulation Boosters
Exercise 4: Legs Up the Wall Pose (Viparita Karani) with Bolster Support
 - Guide expectant mothers through a modified Legs Up the Wall Pose with bolster support to reduce swelling.
 - Discuss the benefits of elevating the legs for improved circulation and fluid drainage.

Exercise 5: Ankle Flex and Point Exercises for Ankle Mobility

- Demonstrate ankle flex and point exercises to enhance ankle mobility and reduce fluid retention.

- Discuss the controlled nature of these movements and their positive impact on circulation.

Exercise 6: Gentle Foot Massage Techniques for Relaxation

- Introduce gentle foot massage techniques to promote relaxation and alleviate swelling.

- Discuss the use of massage techniques such as rolling a tennis ball under the feet for soothing relief.

3. Combating Fatigue: Energizing Sequences for Vitality

Exercise 7: Seated Side Bend and Twist for Midday Rejuvenation

- Guide readers through seated side bends and twists to rejuvenate the body and combat fatigue.

- Discuss the stretching and energizing effects of these movements on the spine and torso.

Exercise 8: Modified Sun Salutations for Gentle Cardiovascular Boost

- Introduce a modified version of Sun Salutations to provide a gentle cardiovascular boost.

- Discuss the importance of controlled movements and breath synchronization for maintaining energy levels.

Exercise 9: Deep Breathing Techniques for Instant Revitalization

- Demonstrate deep breathing techniques, such as diaphragmatic breathing, for instant revitalization.

- Discuss how intentional breathing enhances oxygenation, reduces fatigue, and boosts mental clarity.

4. Adapting Workouts for Each Trimester: Progressive Approaches

Trimester 1: Gentle Introduction to Exercise

- Provide a set of beginner-friendly exercises suitable for the first trimester, focusing on foundational movements.

- Discuss the importance of gradual progression and adapting based on energy levels.

Trimester 2: Building Strength and Flexibility

- Introduce exercises that focus on building strength and flexibility for the second trimester.

- Discuss modifications and variations to accommodate the evolving needs of the body.

Trimester 3: Mindful Maintenance and Preparation for Birth

- Offer exercises for maintaining energy, mobility, and mental well-being during the third trimester.

- Discuss the importance of mindfulness and preparation for the birthing process through specific movements.

By incorporating these targeted exercises and stretches into their routines, expectant mothers can actively address specific challenges associated with pregnancy. Each movement is crafted to provide relief, enhance flexibility, and build strength, empowering women to embrace the transformative journey of pregnancy with resilience and a sense of well-being.

Special Considerations: Workouts for Common Pregnancy Challenges

Section 3: Personal Empowerment - When and How to Modify Exercises Based on Individual Circumstances

Embarking on a fitness journey during pregnancy requires not only dedication but a profound understanding of one's own body. This section serves as a guide, providing insights on when and how to modify or skip certain exercises based on individual circumstances. By empowering expectant mothers with this knowledge, they can tailor their workouts to meet their unique needs, ensuring a safe and enjoyable fitness experience throughout pregnancy.

1. Listening to Your Body: The Key to Individualized Fitness

- Emphasize the importance of tuning into the body's signals during each workout.

- Discuss the role of intuition and self-awareness in recognizing when modifications or skips are necessary.

2. Pregnancy Red Flags: Signs to Modify or Skip Exercises

- Outline common signs and symptoms that may indicate the need for exercise modifications.

- Discuss issues such as dizziness, shortness of breath, pain, or discomfort as cues to adjust the workout.

3.   Consulting   with   Healthcare Professionals: A Preemptive Approach

- Stress the significance of consulting with healthcare professionals before starting or modifying an exercise routine.

- Discuss how personalized advice from healthcare providers ensures a fitness plan aligned with individual health needs.

4. When to Modify: Practical Examples for Common Exercises

Example 1: Squats

- Discuss modifications such as shallower squats or using a stable support for balance.

- Emphasize the importance of maintaining proper form to avoid strain on the lower back and knees.

Example 2: Planks

- Introduce modifications such as inclined planks or performing planks on hands and knees.

- Discuss how these modifications reduce pressure on the abdomen while maintaining core engagement.

Example 3: Cardiovascular Exercises

- Discuss low-impact options such as walking, swimming, or stationary cycling for those experiencing fatigue or joint discomfort.

- Emphasize the adaptability of cardiovascular workouts based on individual energy levels.

5. When to Skip: Cautionary Exercises and Circumstances

Exercise 1: High-Impact Activities

 - Caution against high-impact exercises that may strain the joints and pelvic floor.

 - Discuss alternative low-impact options to protect the body during the various stages of pregnancy.

Exercise 2: Exercises Lying Flat on the Back After the First Trimester

 - Highlight the potential risks of exercises lying flat on the back after the first trimester.

 - Discuss seated or inclined alternatives to maintain comfort and blood circulation.

Exercise 3: Overhead Lifts with Heavy Weights

- Caution against overhead lifts with heavy weights that may strain the lower back.

- Discuss the benefits of using lighter weights and focusing on controlled movements.

6. Crafting a Personalized Fitness Routine: Empowering Expectant Mothers
- Encourage expectant mothers to modify or skip exercises as needed, embracing the principle of self-care.
- Discuss the impact of personalized fitness routines on overall well-being, comfort, and enjoyment.

7. Mindfulness in Motion: The Art of Adaptation

- Introduce the concept of mindfulness in adapting workouts based on individual circumstances.

- Discuss how being present in each movement enhances the mind-body connection, fostering a positive and empowering fitness experience.

By understanding when and how to modify or skip certain exercises based on individual circumstances, expectant mothers can approach their fitness routines with confidence and a keen awareness of their bodies. This mindful approach ensures not only physical well-being but also a positive and enjoyable journey through pregnancy.

Chapter 8

Preparing for Labor and Beyond: The Final Stretch and Postpartum Exercise

Section 1: The Journey to Birth - Exercises for Labor Preparation and Pelvic Floor Health

The final stretch of pregnancy marks a transformative period, a prelude to the momentous event of childbirth. This chapter is dedicated to guiding expectant mothers through exercises specifically designed to prepare the body for labor, with a spotlight on pelvic floor health and endurance. By incorporating these mindful movements, women can embrace the approaching birth with strength, resilience, and a sense of empowered readiness.

1. Understanding the Significance of Labor Preparation Exercises
- Emphasize the role of exercises in preparing the body for the physical demands of labor.
- Discuss the potential benefits, including improved endurance, pelvic floor strength, and overall well-being.

2. Gentle Cardiovascular Workouts for Stamina

Exercise 1: Prenatal Cardiovascular Routine

- Introduce a gentle cardiovascular routine to enhance stamina for labor.

- Discuss low-impact options such as brisk walking or stationary cycling to elevate heart rate gradually.

3. Pelvic Floor Exercises: The Foundation of Labor Readiness
Exercise 2: Kegel Exercises for Pelvic Floor Strengthening

- Guide readers through Kegel exercises to strengthen the pelvic floor muscles.

- Discuss the importance of proper technique and consistency for optimal effectiveness.

Exercise 3: Pelvic Tilts and Circles for Mobility

- Introduce pelvic tilts and circles to promote flexibility and mobility in the pelvic region.

- Discuss how these movements can enhance the body's ability to adapt during labor.

4. Yoga Poses for Labor Preparation
Pose 1: Wide-Legged Child's Pose (Balasana)

- Guide expectant mothers through Wide-Legged Child's Pose to open the pelvic area.

- Discuss the grounding and relaxation benefits of this pose.

Pose 2: Supported Squats (Malasana) for Hip Opening

 - Demonstrate supported squats to encourage hip opening and flexibility.

 - Discuss the supportive elements, such as using props or a stable surface.

Pose 3: Butterfly Pose (Baddha Konasana) for Pelvic Mobility

 - Explore Butterfly Pose to promote pelvic mobility and flexibility.

 - Discuss modifications to accommodate comfort levels and props for added support.

5. Breathing Techniques for Labor and Relaxation

Technique 1: Slow, Deep Belly Breathing

- Introduce slow, deep belly breathing as a technique for relaxation and focus during labor.

- Discuss the calming effects of intentional breathwork in preparation for childbirth.

Technique 2: Patterned Breathing for Coping with Contractions

- Discuss patterned breathing techniques, such as rhythmic inhales and exhales, for coping with contractions.

- Explore the role of breath control in managing pain and maintaining composure.

6. Partner-Assisted Exercises for Labor Support

Exercise 4: Partner-Assisted Squats

- Discuss partner-assisted squats as a collaborative exercise for labor preparation.

- Emphasize communication and support between partners during the movements.

Exercise 5: Pelvic Tilts with Partner Assistance

- Introduce pelvic tilts with partner assistance to enhance pelvic mobility.

- Discuss the shared experience and connection fostered through these exercises.

7. Postpartum Exercise: Nurturing the Body After Birth

- Transition the discussion to postpartum exercise considerations.

- Emphasize the importance of gradual re-entry into physical activity, respecting the body's recovery process.

8. Gentle Postpartum Exercises for Recovery

Exercise 6: Postpartum Pelvic Floor Exercises

- Guide postpartum mothers through gentle pelvic floor exercises to aid recovery.

- Discuss modifications and considerations for the postpartum period.

Exercise 7: Diaphragmatic Breathing for Relaxation

- Introduce diaphragmatic breathing as a calming practice postpartum.

- Discuss the role of intentional breathwork in promoting relaxation and stress relief.

9. Mindful Movement for Postpartum Well-Being

Exercise 8: Postpartum Yoga Sequences for Rejuvenation

- Guide postpartum mothers through gentle yoga sequences for physical and mental rejuvenation.

- Discuss the adaptability of postpartum yoga to accommodate energy levels and physical recovery.

10. Celebrating the Postpartum Journey

- Conclude the chapter by celebrating the postpartum journey as a period of healing, adaptation, and self-care.
- Emphasize the importance of self-compassion and embracing the evolving nature of postpartum well-being.

By delving into these exercises and practices, expectant mothers can not only prepare their bodies for the rigors of labor but also foster a positive mindset and physical resilience for the postpartum period. The final stretch of pregnancy becomes a holistic and empowering journey, laying the foundation for a strong, confident entry into the beautiful realm of motherhood.

Preparing for Labor and Beyond: The Final Stretch and Postpartum Exercise

Section 2: Nurturing Recovery - Gentle Postpartum Workout Routine

Welcoming a new life into the world is a profound experience, and the postpartum period calls for gentle care and intentional recovery. This section offers a tailored postpartum workout routine, designed to aid recovery, rebuild strength, and promote overall well-being. Each exercise is crafted with consideration for the unique needs of postpartum bodies, ensuring a gradual and nurturing return to physical activity.

1. Postpartum Recovery: A Mindful Approach

- Emphasize the importance of approaching postpartum workouts with mindfulness and self-compassion.

- Discuss the gradual nature of recovery, respecting individual timelines and comfort levels.

2. Warm-Up: Gentle Movements to Activate Muscles

Movement 1: Seated Shoulder Rolls

- Guide postpartum mothers through seated shoulder rolls to release tension.

- Emphasize gentle, controlled movements to warm up the upper body.

Movement 2: Ankle Circles for Joint Mobility

- Introduce ankle circles to promote joint mobility and circulation.

- Discuss the benefits of ankle mobility in preparing for weight-bearing exercises.

3. Core Activation: Reconnecting with the Abdominal Muscles

Exercise 1: Pelvic Tilts in Supine Position

- Guide postpartum mothers through pelvic tilts in a supine position to engage the core.

- Discuss the importance of controlled movements to activate abdominal muscles.

Exercise 2: Modified Leg Raises for Lower Abdominal Activation

- Demonstrate modified leg raises to target the lower abdominal muscles.

- Discuss variations and adjustments based on individual comfort and strength.

4. Strengthening the Pelvic Floor: Kegel Exercises

Exercise 3: Seated Kegel Exercises with Breath Coordination

- Guide postpartum mothers through seated Kegel exercises with coordinated breath.

- Discuss the role of Kegels in promoting pelvic floor strength and stability.

5. Lower Body Toning: Gentle Exercises for Strength

Exercise 4: Seated or Standing Marching

- Introduce seated or standing marching to engage the lower body.

- Discuss variations based on comfort and the gradual progression from seated to standing.

Exercise 5: Bodyweight Squats with Support

- Demonstrate bodyweight squats with support to tone the lower body.

- Discuss the use of stable support for balance and safety.

6. Upper Body Strengthening: Building Shoulder and Arm Endurance

Exercise 6: Seated or Standing Arm Circles

- Guide postpartum mothers through seated or standing arm circles for shoulder mobility.

- Discuss the controlled nature of the movement to enhance endurance.

Exercise 7: Bicep Curls with Light Weights

- Introduce bicep curls with light weights to strengthen the arms.

- Discuss the importance of using manageable weights and focusing on form.

7. Cardiovascular Health: Low-Impact Options

Exercise 8: Seated or Standing Marching with Arm Reach

- Combine marching with gentle arm reaches for a low-impact cardiovascular boost.

- Discuss the adaptability of this exercise to accommodate varying energy levels.

8. Cool Down: Relaxing Stretches for Flexibility

Stretch 1: Seated Forward Fold

- Guide postpartum mothers through a seated forward fold to stretch the spine and hamstrings.

- Discuss the importance of breath awareness during the stretch.

Stretch 2: Seated or Standing Chest Opener

- Introduce a seated or standing chest opener stretch for upper body flexibility.

- Discuss the gentle opening of the chest and shoulders.

9. Mindful Breathing: Closing the Routine with Calmness
Breathing Exercise: Diaphragmatic Breathing in Resting Pose

- Conclude the routine with diaphragmatic breathing in a resting pose.

- Discuss the calming and centering effects of intentional breathwork.

By incorporating this gentle postpartum workout routine into their recovery journey, new mothers can embrace physical activity with a focus on healing, strength-building, and overall well-being. This mindful approach ensures a nurturing transition back to exercise, fostering a positive and empowered postpartum experience.

Preparing for Labor and Beyond: The Final Stretch and Postpartum Exercise

Section 3: Gradual Reintegration - Emphasizing Individualized Postpartum Exercise Timelines

Postpartum recovery is a unique and personal journey, and the reintroduction of exercise should align with individual needs and timelines. This section underscores the significance of a gradual approach, emphasizing the importance of honoring one's body and respecting the diverse experiences that come with postpartum recovery. By understanding the individualized nature of this process, new mothers can embark on their fitness journey with patience, self-compassion, and a holistic view of well-being.

1. The Individualized Nature of Postpartum Recovery

- Acknowledge that postpartum recovery varies from person to person.

- Discuss the diverse experiences new mothers may encounter, both physically and emotionally.

2. Listening to Your Body: The Foundation of Postpartum Exercise

- Emphasize the crucial role of listening to one's body during the postpartum period.

- Discuss the significance of tuning into signals of fatigue, discomfort, or readiness for physical activity.

3. Postpartum Fitness as a Personal Journey

- Encourage new mothers to view postpartum fitness as a personal and evolving journey.

- Discuss how the approach to exercise may change over time and adapt to individual recovery timelines.

4. The Role of Hormones in Postpartum Exercise

- Explore the impact of hormonal fluctuations on energy levels and physical readiness.

- Discuss how hormonal changes can influence exercise preferences and intensity during the postpartum period.

5. Gradual Reintegration: A Step-by-Step Approach

Step 1: Focus on Gentle Movements

- Discuss the importance of starting with gentle movements, such as walking or light stretching.

- Emphasize the role of these activities in promoting blood circulation and easing back into physical activity.

Step 2: Core Engagement and Pelvic Floor Exercises

- Introduce core engagement and pelvic floor exercises as foundational components.

- Discuss the gradual incorporation of these exercises to rebuild strength in the abdominal and pelvic areas.

Step 3: Low-Impact Cardiovascular Exercise

- Guide new mothers in adding low-impact cardiovascular exercises, such as swimming or stationary cycling.

- Discuss the cardiovascular benefits and the joint-friendly nature of these activities.

Step 4: Progressive Strength Training

- Introduce progressive strength training with an emphasis on proper form and controlled movements.

- Discuss the gradual increase in resistance and intensity based on individual comfort levels.

6. Postpartum Support: Building a Network of Understanding

- Encourage new mothers to seek support from healthcare professionals, fitness experts, and fellow mothers.

- Discuss how a supportive network can provide guidance, reassurance, and a sense of camaraderie.

7. Patience and Self-Compassion: Essential Elements of Postpartum Exercise
- Stress the importance of patience and self-compassion throughout the postpartum fitness journey.
- Discuss how understanding and embracing the body's natural timeline fosters a positive and empowering experience.

8. Adapting to Changing Circumstances: The Postpartum Fitness Mindset

- Highlight the need for flexibility in the approach to postpartum fitness.

- Discuss how adjustments may be necessary based on factors such as sleep patterns, baby's needs, and emotional well-being.

9.   Celebrating   Small   Victories: Acknowledging Progress

- Encourage new mothers to celebrate small victories and milestones in their postpartum fitness journey.

- Discuss the positive impact of acknowledging progress, no matter how incremental.

By emphasizing the importance of gradually reintroducing exercise postpartum and considering individual recovery timelines, new mothers can navigate their fitness journey with a sense of empowerment and self-awareness. This approach not only prioritizes physical well-being but also fosters a positive mindset, promoting a holistic and sustainable postpartum recovery experience.